# TABLE FOR ONE

*A Life's Journey*

ROBERT VAN HORN

authorHOUSE®

AuthorHouse™
1663 Liberty Drive, Suite 200
Bloomington, IN 47403
www.authorhouse.com
Phone: 1-800-839-8640

First published by AuthorHouse 12/10/2007

ISBN: 978-1-4343-3908-9 (sc)

Printed in the United States of America
Bloomington, Indiana

This book is printed on acid-free paper.

# TABLE OF CONTENTS

# (1) REASSIGNMENT

I cannot begin to tell you when it started I believe it was sometime during the process of obtaining mutual goal of building a nice home in the country where we could raise our four daughters, eventually pay off the mortgage, and retire comfortably. However in between building and living, there, were few short years when we forgot how to communicate and listen. Don't get me wrong, now, we still had a lot of good times. Unfortunately, though, human nature tends to remember the bad more so than the good.

Sometime around March of 1997, we agreed upon a trial separation. I believe we were both emotionally traumatized once the reality of our decision hit us. I called my parents and asked if they would put me up for a while. Of course they agreed. My sister, who lived a mile or so away, wanted me to stay with her and her husband, also. I flip-flopped back and forth for a couple weeks until she called and asked if I wanted to come home. Of course I was overwhelmed with joy, thinking that this nightmare was finally over, and I replied, "I'll be there in an hour or so." I was so excited; I rushed home to greet my family.

Things went great for a few months or so, then all the old aggravations reappeared, and I allowed myself to become angry over the petty problems and differences, which I permitted to irritate me. Good turned into bad in a short amount of time, and before I knew it, I was asked to leave I couldn't believe I allowed the foundation to crumble again.

The plan was set: she and the girls were going out of town for the weekend, and while they were gone, I would move out, hopefully saving the children from some amount of pain. My parents came over to help me move. We loaded some of my belongings, took a short drive down the road to the apartment complex, and began to unload and try to settle in. During the unpacking process, my mind was already working on how to reconcile the marriage. I was not willing to give up eighteen years of marriage without a fight. My goal at this point in my life was to make this woman fall in love with me again. I was going to make this happen or die trying.

My first week in the apartment went fairly smooth. I began to reflect on what percent I was of the problem. Began to take a good, long look at myself, noticed a few things that I didn't particularly care for about myself, and called her one evening and told her what I had discovered about myself and how I was going to change it. Every conversation I had with her during the two years I lived in my apartment, I clutched at every hopeful word I ever heard from her voice, and I prayed for reconciliation. All I could think about at this point in my life was how I wanted my family and my high school sweetheart back. I became somewhat of a nuisance to my family, especially my sister. I would call her after a conversation with my wife and ask her opinion on what was said. After months of this same behavior with no positive responses from anyone I spoke to, it became apparent that I might be beating a dead horse. But my stubborn disposition would not give in.

I became somewhat consumed with alcohol. Each evening, when I returned home from work, I began drinking my six-to-twelve beers. This seemed to ease the pain for a short time, but unfortunately, it was only temporary. I figured I needed to increase the dosage, so on some nights, I consumed eighteen beers. However, after drinking that many beers and feeling the pain of loneliness all around me, I would reach out to my family. They, of course, observed slurring of words, delayed response time, and all other aspects of inebriation. After this had gone on for a month or so, my parents invited me over for a barbecue at their house. Sitting there, waiting for me, was my brother and my two sisters. My family was showing their concern for me by having an intervention. I told them that I would get everything in check, and had no reason for concern any longer. They all had a skeptical look about them. Of course I took their concerns to heart and planned on curtailing my drinking, but the pain was overwhelming I would open the door to the cave of loneliness—those four walls that I was forced to call home. My apartment consisted of four rooms, and within those four rooms there was a bed, recliner, a TV, and a VHS player. After residing in a 2500 square foot home located on two acres, then moving to a 500 square foot apartment I felt slightly claustrophobic.

I began to pay child support immediately. Thoughts on that subject were as follows If I didn't pay it and it ended up in divorce, ultimately I would have to pay it in the end. If this ordeal didn't end up in divorce, then it would show that I was a loving father and had accepted my responsibilities as a parent. In the back of my mind, it occurred to me that this might be something that would help reconcile the marriage, but the subject of reconciliation never seemed to gain any ground.

It had been around four or five weeks already, and I was seriously dying inside to see my kids. But there was a problem there also: my two oldest daughters did not want anything to do with me, and that cut to the bone. My third daughter was the only one who really wanted to have anything at all to do with me. I arranged it with her mother that I could start picking her up on Fridays and bringing her back on Sundays. Our first weekend together was fantastic, we had fast food Friday night for dinner, I took her out for breakfast taco's Saturday morning, and we grilled out Saturday evening, I was trying to do things outside the house so she wouldn't realize that I did not have a dining-room table to eat upon.

Earlier, we had gone to the grocery store to pick up the items needed for grilling out that evening. This kid loves steak, so steak was on the menu for our evening dinner. We had just finished grilling outside, brought the steaks up, and grabbed the vegetables off the stove when she asked me, "Daddy where are we going to eat?"

Thoughts were rushing through my mind at this time, *what am I going to do?* I told her, "Wait here a second, and I will be right back." I grabbed an ice chest from my closet and drug it into the living room, where I presented it to her as my formal dining-room table. We both laughed it off, but I could see the pain in her eyes. We finished dinner and settled in to watch a movie for the evening.

We went to church the next morning, returned to the apartment, and just hung out the rest of the day. We both were enjoying the time that we were spending with each other. We were both watching the clock, trying not to let the other one see, because we were cherishing every moment we were able to spend together, until it was time to take her home. As we walked down the stairs to the parking lot, I had the most gut-wrenching feeling in my stomach that I had ever endured. This was, at the time, the worst feeling I had ever experienced. I tried to lighten the situation by calling her attention to things we passed along the way, but she seemed subdued. When we reached the halfway point, I glanced over and saw tears running down her cheek. This was all I could take. I started crying. She noticed I was crying, and this just intensified her agony. We finally made it back to her house, hugged, cried, said I love you, and told her I would pick her up next week. That gave both of us something to look forward to.

I cried all the way home, and even more when I entered the cave of loneliness. This seemed like a good time to have a couple of beers, but as usual, it only made the situation worse. All I could think about was how much I love all of my children, and how much I wished that I could spend a weekend with all of them like this. As I settled into another evening of depression, I thought, *Well maybe I can call her. That will make me feel better.* I called, and on this occasion, one of the older two answered the phone. Ecstatic at the chance to talk to her, I asked how her day was. She held the phone away from her ear and yelled, "Jessica! It's your father!" I felt like I had been hit by a truck! Words cannot describe what that feels like. It is the most crushing feeling you can ever imagine. I had to put it beside me, though, so that I could talk to Jessica and sound all cheery and happy. The comment made by my older daughter made me realize that I had to, somehow, in some way, regain their love and respect.

Now, I am making no claim to have been the greatest husband or father in the world. In fact, I have made quite a few mistakes in my life. One of the biggest mistakes I have ever made was trying to raise daughters the way my father raised me. That was a huge mistake; one that I take full blame for. But I believe I have mended that situation with three out of four children. I'm still working on the other one—she's a little hardheaded and stubborn, like her daddy.

The Christmas season was slowly approaching us. In the back of my mind, I was thinking, *It's Christmastime She's going to have to want me back now. After all, I have been trying like hell. She's bound to have noticed that.* I was wrong, but I was invited to the in-laws" for Christmas dinner. Of course that sparked some hope in my diminished capacity. I presented the children with their gifts. The stubborn one avoided me, to the point of being flagrantly obvious about it. Her grandfather corrected her, and this at least gave me the opportunity to tell my daughter, "Merry Christmas." I only stayed a short while, but at least I didn't leave depressed—although I probably had a few reasons to be depressed. Money was running low and I was unable to get my children the gifts that I really wanted to give them, but I was thankful for what I was able to do.

At the beginning of the New Year, I decided to change my appearance drastically. I had always had a small problem keeping my weight down, so I joined a health club and started dieting hard. I was making headway in leaps and bounds. When I attended one of Jessica's volleyball games one evening, she informed me that her mother had asked if I had lost weight. Of course I saw that as her noticing me, and that had to be a positive thing, so I kept up the good work. I was quite proud of myself for a while; All my family members had noticed the physical and mental metamorphosis. Easter came along, and Jessica and I traveled to my parents' house. I believe this was the first holiday I got to spend with her alone, so we both knew it would be a good one.

My father had been trying to shake a cold with a hacking cough for a couple of months now. None of us thought too much about it. We just figured he had a common cold. He was diagnosed with lung cancer a few days later. I cried out,"God what have I done that is so terribly wrong?"  Here I am, practically going through a divorce, recovering from a massive stroke myself, alienated from my children, and now, my father is diagnosed with lung cancer?" I said,"Dear God, how much more can I take?"

A few short weeks later, on Sunday morning, Father's day, around eight o'clock a.m., my phone rang. It was one of my dad's friends calling from the hospital to let me know my dad had passed away. Jessica was with me. I was too distraught to call my kids, so I asked her to do it, not realizing at the time how much pressure I was putting on this ten-year-old girl. She made the call though, just like the trooper she's always been. We quickly dressed and went to the hospital.

So here I was faced with more emotional trauma and the only thing I could think of at the time was that the good Lord does not give you a cross that you cannot bear. But I kept thinking to myself, "Lord, this is too much. I cannot bear this burden." I began to pray and as I prayed I felt comfort. Here I was, the oldest sibling,, dealing with four extremely traumatic situations going on in my life at the same time. Obviously I had no answers for what was going on in my life prayer seemed to be the only form of comfort I could find. I was bound and determined not to forsake my wedding vows during this time of separation. Therefore that left me with two things: prayer and Jessica.

I worked and thought diligently about different things we could do during our short weekends together. I pondered, "How can I make an everyday event or chore exciting?"

My quest started out one bright, Saturday morning at an automatic carwash. Jessica was seated in the passenger seat. I watched the spray arm move down my side, and as soon as it turned to travel from driver to passenger side across vehicle rear, I pressed the button to roll her window down. I was busy watching the spray arm's travel, calculating window closing time in my head, and peripherally watching her struggle to remedy her situation. She was shrieking, "DAD! DAD! We are going to get soaked!" My timing was nothing short of perfect; her window was up and sealed a millisecond before water exploded over the entire surface. She looked at me in utter amazement and exclaimed. "That was pretty close, Dad!" From that moment on, opening a window inside a carwash was an anticipated event. On other occasions, I would give her window a little jolt while the spray arm was pointing directly at her window, which caused some squirming and squealing, until she realized she was dry.

With that errand taken care of, now is the time to relieve myself of the bothersome chore of grocery shopping. As we entered a local store, my devious mind was going a mile a minute. "What can I do in here to freak her out?" We were casually traversing each aisle in search of needed goods, when it finally hit me: I requested she push our cart, then hurried in front of her, quickly looked both directions, then performed a ballerina's pirouette in middle of aisle. I then looked in her direction—she was crouching behind our cart, looking in all directions, to make sure nobody saw me. She stood up, shot a grin in my direction, called me a dork, and said, "You would be pretty embarrassed if anybody saw you do that! To this day, she tells me, "Behave in the grocery store!"

My weekends with Jessica were the most precious assets I had at the time. I cherished every moment we spent together, and I wanted every moment she spent with me to be filled with excitement and fun. We made it a Saturday-morning ritual to go out for breakfast tacos. This particular weekend, I was, for lack of a better word, broke. Both of us had cleaned up and dressed Saturday morning when she asked, "What kind of tacos are you going to eat this morning, Dad?" I was frantic. I didn't want to tell her we would have to break tradition because I was broke. I replied, "I'm not very hungry today." I hoped she would say the same, but of course she replied, "I'm starving!" Thoughts were rushing through my head. *What am I going to do? Do I have any cash stashed in my truck? No wait, my change jar!* I hurriedly grabbed it and counted about three dollars in change. My mind eased. This would be enough for her; I just wouldn't eat, so off we went. After standing in line for a minute or so, I asked her what she wanted. She told me and I asked her to get us a table, because I would be there in a minute. I didn't want her to see me paying with change or to have to explain why I did not order. I placed the order, then went to sit with her. We were talking for a couple of minutes when they called our number. I requested that she get the condiments of her choice, and I would get the tray. I was still trying to avoid questions. When we sat and she saw I had nothing, she asked why. I replied, "Remember, I'm not very hungry." She was very smart and saw right through me. Knowing something was up; she said "I'm not as hungry as I thought. Why don't you eat this second taco?" I kept insisting I was not hungry, but all the while, she was insisting I eat. After exhausting my efforts, I finally gave in and told her, "Okay but you're making me go off my diet." She watched me eat every bite, then asked if she could help me with my chores today. I thought, *Lord, you really blessed this one.*

After six months or so, my youngest started joining Jessica and me on weekends. When I first heard of her desire to visit me, I was so thrilled I could hardly control my enthusiasm. I needed to begin planning for two on weekends now. For instance, where was everyone going to sleep? All I had that was mine was a twin bed and a couch my cousin had loaned me. Jessica was too scared to sleep in a different room than me, so I decided to throw the mattress on the living room floor, along with couch cushions, so we would camp out. They absolutely loved it. Obviously, I didn't sleep well like this, but I was willing to endure any type of hardship to be with my children. The next hardship was financial. Somehow now I needed to entertain two instead of one. Whatever it was I did could not have been much, but we still enjoyed our time together. I played games with them, helped Jessica build a cardboard maze for a school project, and made so-called jewelry with Catherine by twisting brass brazing rods together with a cordless drill. We had a blast together!

Just a few short years later, Lindsey started calling and coming around. Her emergence happened one Friday night while I was spending the weekend with a friend of mine at the lake. I was standing outside when my phone rang. Buddy was inside, unaware of my conversation. I did not recognize the number, and I said, "Hello?"

I heard, "Dad?"

"Yes," I replied.

"This is Lindsey."

I was shocked, then worried that something had happened. I asked, "What's going on?"

She replied, "Nothing I just wanted to call and see how you are doing."

We talked for fifteen minutes or so when she informed me that she needed to go. I replied, "It was nice talking to you."

Then she said, "I love you!"

I immediately got all choked up and told her I loved her, too, and I missed her dearly. She said goodbye, and I started to cry. I had been working on this kid for what seemed an eternity. Buddy came outside saw my tears and wanted to know what was going on. I told him what had happened, and then I exclaimed, "I got another one back!"

He doesn't have children, but he could understand my tears were tears of joy.

My duration in the cave of loneliness had exceeded a year now, with no changes looming on the horizon. One evening, I had a little extra cash on me, and I decided to treat myself to dinner. Extra cash was not a common occurrence those days, and I had wanted to try a Mexican food restaurant located nearby. I walked inside, stood and waited for the hostess. She approached, cheerfully greeted me, and asked, "Table for two?"

I replied, "No, just one!"

This stuck in my mind like a spike in a rail, and it also inspired my book title. After I was seated, my waitress approached. Before reaching my table, I noticed her nametag. She had the same name as my ex-wife, which is an uncommon name. I had only known one other person besides my ex-wife with this name. I thought, *Here I am, trying to enjoy one of life's simple pleasures, and I get a reminder of my situation.* I finished my meal and went home to settle in for a Seinfeld episode. George was reporting to Jerry about a new restaurant he had visited. Jerry asked who accompanied him. George replied, "I went by myself!" Jerry started criticizing George by telling him how much he resembled a loser for dining alone. My thoughts were: *Oh, brother, what else do I need to remind me of this situation?*

Sometime around early spring of the year 2000, we met at my attorney's office. My attorney and I walked into a conference room where she sat with her attorney. I could feel my stomach rising into my throat. I was thinking, *How could two intelligent people who cared for each other let it come to this?* My mind continued to struggle with these questions while our respective attorneys haggled back and forth over the division of property, which seemed to have no degree of significance at the time. My mind was racing back and forth. *How can I put a stop to this?* I found no solutions.

A few short weeks later, I received a call from my attorney's office, letting me know that they were just served with divorce papers. My heart sank, and my eyes welled with tears. I began to feel the most unbelievable pain and anguish I had ever experienced in my life. I had questions to answer, so I need to quickly regain my composure. For instance: when was a good time for me to come in review the decree and sign? I set up an appointment with them, went in, reviewed the decree with my attorney, asked him to resolve an issue I did not agree with, and then signed. I left that office a shell of the man I used to be. I told my children when this all started that I would fight for reconciliation to the bitter end, and that they could put that on my headstone one day. I believe I fulfilled the promise I made to my children. I guess I could have refused to sign and dragged it out longer, but if she was willing to take it this far, then obviously, there was no turning back. It was time for each of us to get on with our lives. My only regret was that I failed to do more earlier on in the marriage. She's a wonderful woman and mother, and deserves all the happiness life can bring her.

My advice on this subject is: "If you can avoid the misery divorce brings, then avoid it like the plague." The covenant of marriage is sacred and should not be taken lightly.

# (2) READJUST

I mentioned in the previous chapter that I was recovering from a stroke. This occurred October 20, 1995, just three weeks after my thirty-sixth birthday. I was milling around in the twelve-hundred-square-foot workshop that I had built and been diligently attempting to complete. I had only to complete all the wiring to have a finished product. I had some extension cords running from an outlet on the power pole outside to provide temporary power. I was ready to relax and listen to a High School football game. The radio was tuned in, and I sat down in my chair, ready for some gridiron action. My doctor had recently changed my arrhythmia medication, and had informed me it might make me feel weak. All of a sudden, I unwillingly slid out of my chair, onto the floor. Unbeknownst to me, I had just suffered a stroke. Bewildered and a little dazed and confused, I tried to push myself up from the floor. My left arm was of little use as I thought to myself, *Well, she told me this new medication might make me feel weak, but this is ridiculous.* I managed somehow to make it to my feet, but not for long. I plummeted to the concrete floor, face-first, receiving a black eye, accompanied by a concussion. I'm not sure, but I believe this rendered me unconscious for a short period of time. After I awoke, I began trying to drag myself toward the overhead door, possibly to call for help. My two youngest were inside the house, watching television; maybe I could get their attention. But I had another obstacle hidden in my path—I was swinging my right arm out in front of me, pulling with it and pushing with my right leg. I swung my arm in front of me again, only to land on a frayed extension cord where I received a heck of an electrical shock. I managed to remove myself from the hazard. Exhausted and confused, I decided to wait until somebody found me.

I do not know how long I laid on the floor, waiting for help. My wife returned home from volleyball practice with the oldest two and asked the younger two where I was. They responded, "Out in the workshop." Keep in mind, there were no lights on inside my shop. She walked in, found me on the floor, and began asking questions. I guess, from my slurred speech, she ascertained that I'd had a stroke. She said, "I'll be right back, I'm going to call nine-one-one."

Lindsey came out and sat with me while the paramedics were summoned. I was rushed to the hospital, where they performed the usual barrage of medical tests and procedures. My wife had called my parents, and they rushed in. They lived about an hour outside San Antonio. After reviewing the MRI, the neurologists informed my wife and parents that the damage was so severe, he had no hope I would ever walk again. At this point in time, I was classified as a hemiplegic, as my whole left side was non responsive. The gravity of the situation hit me, and I knew I was in for a heck of a fight. When the neurologists informed me that he had no hope that I would ever walk again, my colorful response to him was, as follows: "Bull! Watch me." This was the beginning of a two-week stay at this hospital, where I underwent the usual barrage of tests, the pain of physical therapy, and the mental anguish of not knowing what life had in store for me.

Finally, the day came when they had taken me as far as they could take me, and it was time to go to a rehabilitation facility, where I underwent the most strenuous work I'd ever done in my life. It's extremely difficult for people who've never been in this situation before to understand and to try to cope with the unknown variables you're dealing with, but my wife and children were by my side the whole time. The mental anguish of gazing daily upon a semi-lifeless arm and leg was excruciating. My father had recently retired and was spending most of his day with me at rehab. I could see mental torment upon his face as I struggled with performing simple motor-skill tasks, such as attempting to pick something up, then placing it on a higher shelf. I went to occupational and physical therapy daily, where I would attempt to perform basic motor skills, like extending my arm or lifting my leg. I was bound and determined to regain my mobility and put an end to this perpetual nightmare. Following my session with a therapist, I would return to my room and perform the same exercises that I had just performed with the therapist.

I had reached a point in my therapy where I was capable of some limited movement within my room. I had come a long way, but I had a long way to go.

I decided to spend my first weekend at rehab in their gym, where I usually do my therapy. I rolled in bright and early Saturday morning, ready to conquer the world on my own. I set up an area to work, removed a pinch tree from the cabinet, and began my therapy, on my own. Any occupational or physical therapist will recognize the term *pinch tree*. For all of you out there unfamiliar with this terminology, allow me to elaborate: a pinch tree is a small, artificial tree with clothes pins attached to different limbs. The object is to extend your arm, pinch a clothes pin, remove it from that limb, and place it on another limb. Sounds pretty easy, doesn't it? Not after having the part of your brain that controls theses functions destroyed. I began struggling with the task at hand, groaning and straining to reach and grasp. After about ten or fifteen minutes, I had managed to move and place two clothes pins. I noticed a man walk in, carrying a five- or six-year-old girl. He began working with her, and after a few minutes of casual observation; I surmised she had suffered some sort of head injury, also. She was struggling with simple tasks, also. I continued my workout and watched her out of the corner of my eye. Her struggles were tearing me up inside. I began to weep profusely as I felt this small child's pain. I guess she noticed me and asked, "Daddy why is that man crying?"

He replied, "I'm not sure, sweetheart, maybe he just doesn't feel well!"

This just elevated my anguish, which increased the difficulty of my therapy. I cried out inside, "Lord, please give me her pain! I can handle it much better than this innocent child can. Please, Lord, let me have her pain,. By this time, I was almost sobbing, fearing my sobbing might upset her progress. I decided I'd had enough for one day, so I replaced the pinch tree, shot them a smile, and said, "Keep up the good work." Then I rolled myself back to my room.

I never saw the little girl again, but I often wondered what her outcome was! Sometimes I wondered if she was an angel sent by God to tell me: "If a little girl can fight with all she's got, then so can you." I like to believe she was an angel!

A simple task like buttoning your shirt, tying your shoes, or squeezing toothpaste onto your toothbrush were some of the most arduous tasks I had to attempt on a daily basis. I spent approximately three weeks in rehab and around two months in outpatient rehab. I had not reached full recovery, and the doctors said it could take up to a year to regain more, and after that, I would regain nothing else. I can remember praying day and night while in rehab, begging the Lord to hear my prayers. I was showing him my willingness to fight, and I was asking him for some help with the fight. He showed me unconditional mercy.

I remember waking one morning, a day that I was due for outpatient therapy, and thinking to myself that something was different, but I didn't know at the time what was different. I stretched my arms out and yawned and unknowingly spread my fingers on my left hand. This was something I had not been able to do since the stroke. I could open my hand and grasp objects, but I could not spread my fingers apart. When I arrived for rehab, I hastily searched for my occupational therapist. Brimming with joy, I told her, "Check this out!" You would have thought she had won the lottery. It was difficult to believe her degree of enthusiasm and joy over this simple task. I would often amuse the hospital staff by walking in, and instead of using the cane they gave me; I would carry it on my shoulder. Later on that day, I had an appointment with my neurologist, who had not seen me since I left the hospital. I was sitting in his waiting room when he came out of the back and called my name. I stood up and walked into the examination room, he had this bewildered look on his face, and I asked, "What's the matter? Are you surprised to see me?"

He replied, "I thought I would see you again, but thought that you would be in a wheelchair." Of course, in disbelief, he had to check every aspect of my mobility and strength, and he was totally astonished at the recovery. I told him I had done nothing but try—God did the rest.

I really didn't want to get that long-winded on the subject of the stroke, but I thought it was imperative that you know my physical, mental, and psychological status at the time I was dealing with an impending divorce, the loss of my father, and alienation from my children. I began to feel sorry for myself, and I started drinking heavily. We all know how difficult life can be. I found myself falling into a rut, and self pity had me pinned to the mat like a professional wrestler. The daily pain of returning to the cave of loneliness was overwhelming at times. The only refuge I seemed to find was in the voice of my daughter. Just talking to her made many of my troubles and cares fade. And even after receiving harsh criticism from an older sibling due to her involvement with me, she remained steadfast and loyal. She was quite an individual, and has turned out to be an unbelievable young lady. She has stood by my side ever since I had to leave the house, and she continues to remain there today.

# (3) REBOUND

As in most cases when human nature is involved, a rebound is inevitable. This, of course, happened to me. I met her a few months after the divorce was final, when my level of vulnerability was probably at its highest. I was gullible and responsive to anyone showing the slightest bit of interest. This girl was totally wrong for me, but she seemed to say all the right things—words that I needed to hear at the time. We began to see each other on a fairly regular basis. It appeared that, no matter what type of environment we were in, we always managed to have a really good time. I was becoming caught in a web of mistruths and deceit, but I was so infatuated at the time, I merely overlooked these facts and played them off as coincidence. I begin to think that I was acquiring some really true feelings for this girl, so I decided to continue with the dating process, get to know more about her, and not be so quick to condemn. Basically, I overlooked the obvious and continued my quest for happiness. We continued to go out to different places and have a great time. It almost seemed like she was a dream come true. This girl was really becoming something that I cared for and was beginning to trust.

On one occasion we went to Austin, just to hang out, drive around, and see different sites. We ended up at a restaurant that hosted a band playing a lot of sixties and seventies rock. It was a really fun experience: I was in good company, listening to good music, and had a wonderful dinner in front of me. I thought I was in heaven. We returned to our respective homes that evening and met at a local lake the next morning for some jet-ski fun in the sun.

I began slowly to introduce her to members of my family. She first met my mother and me for dinner one evening. My mother was also taken by her charm. She seemed so irresistible and charming. How could I question her peculiar answers to questions and strange behavior patterns? It was impossible for me to believe that she could be deceiving me in any way, shape, or form. I dismissed it as distrust on my part—here I was taking the blame again. But I did not blame myself for long. On another occasion, a comparable instance happened, similar to what had previously happened before, and this time she had a different excuse. I wasn't going to take it sitting down this time. I wanted an explanation, and an explanation was all that would satisfy my curiosity! The explanation she gave was so farfetched and twisted, I ended up throwing my hands up and saying, "That's it, I can't take anymore!" I guess you can say that self-preservation kicked in, and I had to get out of this thing before I got hurt again. My only advice regarding this subject is: CAUTION.

I look back on this period of my life at times and regard it as filling a void in my life that needed to be filled. Thank God nothing more ever became of this. I often reflect on how my eyes were so closed and dimmed by the words that I thought I needed to hear. I also believe that this was just preparing me for the one who was going to be my world and my life. Shortly after ending this relationship I began to look online, just out of curiosity. I met and talked to a few women whom I was attracted to, and I tried starting slowly. It was just your average question-and-answer session, but I never got to meet any women that I was really attracted to. They always seemed to get spooked before it came time to meet. This erratic behavior seemed to be very common throughout all of the personals available. I had viewed and researched almost every personal available online.

I switched my account from one to another and ended up with the one that I have today.

The summer of 2004 was spent searching the personals column, and I found one who looked to be heaven-sent. She didn't live too far away from me—just a little bit southwest of Austin. I attempted to make contact, but her profile showed that she had not been active in months. I continued writing her anyway, and five long months went by before she responded. She just made a casual response, though; nothing that showed any type of interest. I couldn't believe it. I had met all of her criteria except, for one thing: I was not a college graduate. My stubborn self continued on for another year or so. I thought that, if I got a response out of her, maybe I could say something in one of my letters that would break the ice somewhat. Frustration finally set in, and I basically said in my final letter to her, "Life is too short." Obviously she wasn't interested. I can understand that, but at least she could let me know. For some reason or another, I wanted to hear from her, but she was not interested. Then I received a quick response from her. Of course it was not a favorable response, but at least now I knew exactly where I stood.

Another occasion prior to this, on Christian personals, I met a woman whom I contacted after finding out we both went to the same high school. I thought, "Wow, what a great start! Lots in common, no big age difference, we ought to be able to relate on the same plane." We began chatting back and forth for several weeks. This was looking extremely promising, and she didn't live far from me. I would rush home daily to read mail from her. Everything was going great, and it was time to mention a meeting of some sort. The day I planned to request a meeting, I arrived home hurriedly, logged onto the site, and read my mail. To my total shock and surprise, I read, "Stop writing my wife, you /*& #@ % !&%*#." This was obviously a bad sign. I never logged onto that site again.

These few strokes of bad luck did not deter me in my quest. I was bound and determined to find my soul mate. I just knew she existed within the confines of one of these personals sites, so my search continued, believing wholeheartedly that this site would produce the woman of my dreams—a woman whose undying love for me would prevail through thick and thin; a woman who was truly, madly, deeply in love with me. I knew she existed, because one night, while deep in prayer, I received an answer. The answer was, "I have someone special picked out for you, but you will have to be patient, because it will take a long time. When it happens, everything will be wonderful." The words *ten years* kept echoing in my mind. I thought, "Dear God, please don't tell me it's going to take ten years!" Looking back, I now understand why this process was taking so long. First of all, people don't change overnight. The changes that had occurred in my life over the past ten years were a testimonial to my spiritual growth. I had seen remarkable changes in my life, my thoughts, ,my priorities, and my temperament—all of which were for the better.

I paid a visit to my former and recently retired pastor. He and his wife cheerfully greeted me at their door and invited me in for some iced tea. His wife, knowing I was divorced, asked if I had found a girlfriend yet. I replied, "No, all is still silent on that front." Then I remarked, "A couple of friends took me to a club a few weeks back, and I never felt so out of place in my life."

She replied, "You're not going to find a quality woman in a bar!"

I responded, "I know, I was just curious what all the hoopla was about." Then I told them, "I decided to wait on the Lord, because if I try to push this, it will just end up in headache and heartache."

I became a regular at a local restaurant and sports bar, where all the wait staff were college-age girls. This brought concern from some family members.

They thought I was looking for a wife there, when in actuality, these girls were serving as a surrogate family. It got to where I couldn't walk in without having four or more girls walk up greet and hug me. They had gotten to know me and most of all, trust and respect me. They would ask my advice with problems concerning parents, finances, boyfriends, etc. I would cook food and bring it to the restaurant for them—after all, they were starving college students. A select few were allowed to request food to take home, and they were somewhat reluctant, out of respect for me. After a short amount of time, they became much less hesitant. There are a few I was eternally grateful for; but unfortunately, in today's society, even mentioning a first name could cause some legal ramifications, therefore these pseudonyms will have to suffice: Tigger and Roo, Beavis and Butthead. I want all of you to know your friendship came at a time in my life when I needed it. I am grateful and blessed to have friends who care for me the way all of you did. On one occasion, I revealed to one of the young women the details regarding my stroke. She was in shock and utter amazement at my recovery, then she replied "You must be pretty proud of your accomplishment!" I began to witness to her about how there was no way I could have done this all on my own, that in actuality, God deserves the glory. She began attending church on a regular basis again, and as far as I know, she is still going.

Butthead, you made me laugh so much, I would forget my troubles. Your stories were always hysterical. You are a sweet and caring person. I wish you all the joy and happiness life can bring you, even though you bring happiness everywhere you go!

# (4) RESOURCES

During my travels through the rebound cycle, I decided to start my own business, which is something I had only dreamed of doing before. This was it: my own remodeling business. I was in heaven. Finally, I had accomplished my dream, and I had enough courage to try. The first few months went fairly well. I managed to stay fairly busy; not bad for a man who went into business by word of mouth only. The jobs just kept on rolling in, big and small. I began to build my arsenal of tools required for other jobs. I became more and more diverse, and I had a three-and-a-half-month backlog of work. I couldn't believe how work just kept pouring in. Something in the back of my mind told me that I needed to prepare for slow times. Around October, it began to slow down substantially. I barely had enough business to pay my bills, but I kept plugging away. November came and went with little to no business, and I had to dip into my savings to pay my monthly bills. December was awful, I sat idle most of the month, and that seemed to spill into January and February. I finally picked up enough work to keep me busy through March. Then the phones really started ringing again. Now I was looking at another substantial backlog of work, but the hard times of winter taught me a real lesson. Luckily, I was smart enough the first go-round, and realized that the backlog would not remain, and that I needed to put money away for hard times.

This type of business is usually hot and cold, so preparations for the cold times are a must. I saved a little out of each job for the cold times. I was also enjoying the freedom that self-employment brought—it enabled me to do things personally at times that I did not have the ability to do before. I picked up a patio enclosure, which led to a whole house remodel during the winter months of that year, which sustained me through December. I was feeling confident enough to decide on buying a new truck. This particular weekend, my youngest two were spending the weekend with me. I left to pick up some breakfast for them. Upon my return I told them I had to leave, but would be back shortly. They politely nodded yes while stuffing breakfast tacos in their mouth. I headed up to the local dealership to inquire about price, payment plans, etc. I made the deal and returned home to strip my truck of all toolboxes, etc. On the way home, I conjured up a plan about how to surprise the girls with my new truck. After arriving, I told them I needed their help removing all of the truck's contents, because I needed to help a friend move some big things. They got dressed, came outside, and began helping. Without question, they jumped in at my request to help me move these objects. When I pulled into the dealership, I was hit with a barrage of questions. They were satisfied when I told them I just wanted to inquire about a price. They waited in the truck for me while I was signing papers.

I gave the salesman my keys, and when he went outside to get the truck, he met an ornery fourteen-

and twelve-year-old who loudly proclaimed, "This is my dad's truck, and you better leave it alone!" About this time, I emerged from inside to witness the confrontation. My salesman politely told them that it was no longer my truck, and my truck was the new one sitting next to it. Those two became so ecstatic; they could hardly contain their enthusiasm. They were both so happy for me, it was unbelievable. Of course, Jessica couldn't wait to drive it, so I took her to a friend's property, which was loaded with gravel roads, and I got out and let her go. She was having a blast, but I noticed she kept stopping in these puddles of water, then would take off again. I didn't think much of it, and I let her go another fifteen or twenty minutes. Then I motioned for her to come back. I got in and asked her why she had stopped in all those puddles. She told me she got stuck, but she put it in four-wheel drive and it pulled right on out! I sat there in disbelief. I had not put it in four-wheel drive myself yet. I chuckled to myself and thought, *I didn't nickname her "Wild Thing" as a small child for nothing.*

Business was going pretty well; I was picking up larger jobs that required longer materials and additional tools. My business was growing. I had two full-time helpers and two part-time. I became weary of loading tools and supplies every morning and unloading every evening, so I decided to buy an open-bed trailer. When I mounted my toolbox on the front, I thought, *I'm almost first class now*. Besides, I had just acquired a contract with a local property-management agency that had over a hundred homes. I thanked God for his blessings and started enjoying the steady work and steady income that steady work provides. My help and I were knocking these houses out, one right after another, and having a fairly relaxed time while performing our work.

I checked my list to see which house was next, and I took off to refresh my memory and get another look at the monster. It was a small house, but in dire need of large-scale repair and maintenance. The fence was falling down, half the siding on the house was rotten, and in desperate need of paint inside and out. This was going to take some time. I loaded everything onto the trailer the next morning and struck out to accomplish my work. I met the guys at the house and started chipping away. Four days later, we finished. I had never been so glad to finish a project in my life. Hot, tired, and sweaty, I went home, all the time debating in my mind whether to unload the trailer or mow the lawn. I opted to mow the lawn—after all, I had everything secure on my trailer. The next day, I picked up my two youngest, and we drove around and went shopping, just having fun. We were on the way back to my house around three p.m. I stopped at the stop sign for my street, glanced down toward my house, and my heart sank to my stomach. My trailer was gone. I hurried toward my house, got out, and looked at my driveway, which used to have my trailer and every tool I owned on it. I fought with every ounce of fiber in my body to maintain my composure. I saw a piece of the trailer lock lying on my driveway—it had been cut. The girls were in tears by this time. They both knew how hard I had worked to get this far. I assured them everything was going to be all right, because I thought my homeowner's policy would cover some replacement costs. Boy, was I disillusioned. My homeowner's policy did not cover anything.

I thought, *Dear Lord, what am I going to do? I don't even have a hammer now! Everything is gone.* I began to pray and ask God for guidance, and much to my astonishment, small painting jobs began to flow in. These jobs required only rollers, brushes, etc. These small jobs enabled me to start slowly replacing stolen items. My sister remarked about how well I handled this crisis and how calm I was about the whole thing. She said she would have been devastated if she was placed in that position, and she just couldn't believe how I was handling it. I told her I was blessed and highly favored, and the Lord would provide.

# (5) RECOVERY

My family has been very supportive throughout this ordeal. My mother always told me
as a child, "Your friends will come and go, but when
it comes to people caring, nobody will care like a
family member."

I jumped the gun a little in the previous chapter
and failed to inform you of my home purchase,
right after the divorce was final. I had lots of family
members help me move—after all, I had belongings in two different places: my apartment and my
former home. I had built a twelve-hundred-square-
foot workshop, which housed my collection of tools,
varying from woodworking tools to torches and
welders, all of which had to be relocated to my new

home. It was like trying to pack ten pounds of taters into a five-pound sack, but I got it all in my garage. I bought a few new items, like a couch and loveseat, with my settlement money, but the rest went to bills, attorneys' fees, etc. Oh yes, and I bought my Jet-Ski. I think I bought that item out of spite more than anything else, but I sure had a lot of fun on it. That's one example of how God has changed me into the person I am today. The very thought of a spiteful act doesn't even cross my mind anymore. I sometimes think of how I used to be, and I thank the Lord above for putting me into the fire to remove those impurities. I can't even begin to describe how much better life is now.

Back to the subject of the Jet-Ski…

Since Jessica had always been there for me, she was obviously the first to experience a trip to the lake. I prepared a lunch for the two of us, stowed it onboard, and off we went. We must have traveled the majority of the lake, just enjoying the majestic scenery, when I decided to pull into a cove and swim for a while. Before I could remove the safety lanyard from my wrist, she informed me that she was hungry.

I replied, "Well we can go back to the picnic area to eat or just sit here on the water and enjoy our lunch."

She jumped at the idea of eating lunch while sitting on the ski in the water. During our lunch consumption, we engaged in conversation about different things. Then she commented, "You sure have come a long way since living in that apartment,

I replied, "We sure have, sweetheart. Hasn't God been good to us?"

She agreed, then dove into the water with her lifejacket on and coaxed me in with statements like, "Come on in! The water feels great." We floated and talked for about an hour, and then she was ready for some more high-speed fun.

On another lake trip, we went pretty far across the lake to a lakeside restaurant for lunch. I had stowed some dry clothes for us to wear inside. She thought that was the greatest thing, riding a Jet-Ski to a restaurant, going inside, eating, and watching boaters and water-skiers go by.

My children had begun to notice a change in me, and they commented, "Wow, Dad, you sure are a calm person now."

My second oldest requested that I build her a nightstand like I had built for my oldest. I cheerfully agreed, under one condition, which was I would not work on it alone. She had to be there and help. Everything was agreed upon, and we began our project together. I knew going into this that the project would not be completed quickly, due to her schedule.

I arrived home from church one Sunday morning with my left foot feeling like somebody had run over it with a truck. I didn't know at the time that I had a torn Achilles tendon and heel-spur. I was content in the thought of relaxing at home and doing absolutely nothing. Then my phone rang. It was Lindsey, asking if we could work on her nightstand. Without hesitation, I told her, "Yes, come on over." I was overcome with pain, but I could not disappoint her. After all, it took several years to regain my status with her. Upon her arrival, I informed her of my predicament, letting her know I would not be moving at regular speed. We were assembling pieces together, and I attempted to pull some slack in my cord, but I inadvertently unplugged it. Fearing an outburst on my part, she backed off. I calmly hobbled over, reconnected it, and went back to work. She stared at me in disbelief. I just grinned, even though the pain was crippling at the time. She stayed late, and made and ate dinner with me while we talked about her project and what type of stain and finish she would like to use on it. I believe she decided to stain and finish her nightstand herself, in order to keep me from aggravating my injury any further. She is quite a perceptive individual, wouldn't you say?

Times like those made me realize how much time I lost being aggravated with life. It was stupid and irresponsible. Don't we all wish we could turn back the hands of time and change something in our past?

My first Christmas in my new house was going to be an eventful one. I had gifts under the tree for them and a neat surprise in their stocking and mine. When gift-unwrapping was complete, I told them to check out their stockings. They each reached in and pulled out a small can of silly string. They all had bewildered looks on their faces, and I explained, "Someone's can is empty, and once you figure out whose, then you get them with yours." I opened mine, pointed at the older two, pushed the button and said, "Oh no this one is empty."

All four started shooting me with intermittent shots of string. I produced another can and said, "This one works," and I started covering as many of them as I could get. Immediately, I was hit with string from four directions. Everybody laughed and thought it was the greatest. I was still cleaning small bits of silly string from inside my house several months later.

Jessica and Catherine were weekend regulars at my house, and I had exhausted my efforts of new and exciting things to do with them—that is, until I came up with a brainstorm one day and incorporated bowling and coconuts. They both were an easy sell on the idea, so off we went to purchase coconuts. During our return trip home, all three of us were formulating the rules for the game. Upon arriving at home, we rushed to the backyard where the grass was freshly mowed, eager to get started. Each of use picked a coconut to use as a ball, and I had purchased extras, just in case. We practiced rolling them to get an idea of a desired distance. Keep in mind that rolling an oblong object straight on an irregular surface is no easy task. I proceeded to set six coconuts up in a triangular pattern.

Jessica and Catherine were both anxious to get started. I had already predetermined a rotation schedule of bowling, resetting, and scorekeeping; that way, everyone always had something to do. They were totally engrossed in this game. While we were laughing and cheering each other on, time just flew by. I was ready to reset after Jessica bowled, but her coconut hit the front pin head-on and exploded, drenching me in coconut milk.

Jessica rushed over and asked, "Are you all right?"

I said, "Of course, I just had not planned on a coconut-milk bath."

They both were in hysterics by this time, and we gathered up the broken pieces of coconut and ate them. I looked at Jessica and said, "You did that just so you can eat one, didn't you?" She looked at me with a sheepish grin and said, "Sort of." We resumed play, and I cautioned them to be careful while resetting.

Earlier, Catherine had turned a radio on inside and turned it up loud enough to drown out the doorbell and the knocking coming from the front door. My attention was drawn away as I looked toward my locked gate where my ex-wife was trying to get anyone's attention. She was there to pick up the girls. I unlocked the gate and invited her in, where she began looking around, a little bewildered about what we were doing. Then she asked, "Girls, what are you doing?"

They cheerfully replied, "Coconut Bowling!" Then they began to tell her the object of the game, the rules, etc. My ex-wife then asked, "What do you do if one breaks?"

They replied loudly, "You eat it!" She smiled and told them it was time to go home. I couldn't believe the afternoon had flown by that fast. They began to gather their belongings and load them into their mother's car, and they asked me if we could play that game again next weekend. Of course, I was thrilled about their degree of enthusiasm, and I let them know we could play that game as often as they wished. To this day, I still have half a coconut shell in my house.

# (6) REFLECTIONS

Sometime around four or five years ago, after thinking about it for several months, I decided I needed to switch churches. This was not an easy decision. This church I considered leaving was the one I had been a member of since birth. This revelation came to me one Sunday morning when had I turned on the TV and listened to my future pastor preach. I got so much out of his sermon that morning that I decided this church would be my future home. I began attending the morning services at 8:30 a.m. I was searching for something, I sort of knew, but I really didn't know, in the back of my mind, what I was really looking for. Every sermon I listened to seemed as if it was directed at me. I was at the point in my life where it seemed like everything that was happening in my life had a specific reason. My spiritual life was waking from its slumber, and I was drawing closer to God. God was probably thinking at that moment, "It's about time, dummy." After a few months of attending Cornerstone Church, I knew in my heart I had found my home.

I began to tell my mother I was going to church in order to recharge my batteries. She knew exactly what I meant. My mother seemed quite proud of the path I had now embarked on, and she asked several of her friends and family members, "How many single men do you know that will drag their hind parts out of bed and attend church at 8:30 every Sunday morning?"

Their response was, "Not many!"

My first attendance at Cornerstone was an early one. Not sure of service times, I arrived thirty minutes early and made my way to the front section of pews. The choir was warming up, and then a slender, attractive, forty-ish woman walked out and began singing a song. I thought to myself, *This might be difficult, but I think I can get used to it.* I was so touched and moved by the music ministry and sermon that I knew I was hooked. Shortly thereafter, I began attending the over-forty-singles Sunday school class in hopes of meeting a Godly woman. Obviously my time of waiting had not elapsed. In light of this revelation, I surmised that my relationship with God had not evolved to his prearranged height yet, so I began to focus on myself and what God wanted out of me. I reverted back to attending only church and trying to grow spiritually. This was probably one of the wisest decisions I have ever made.

One Sunday morning during our music ministry, I noticed an attractive woman sitting a few pews in front of me. She began to raise her hands and praise God. It was that moment in time when I realized what I wanted in a woman. I prayed a quick little prayer, asking the Lord for a woman who could raise her hands in praise like this one. Earlier in my church life, I found it difficult to raise my hands in praise. I suffered from this difficulty for a little less than a year at Cornerstone, but then I realized that raising my hands is a submissive act that should be performed frequently.

Early in my life at Cornerstone, on my way to church one Sunday morning, my heart was heavy. I was becoming angry with life. Was suffering from loneliness, business was slow to non-existent, and subsequently, my bills were piling up, I felt as if the weight of the world was on my shoulders. I quickly found a seat and began to pray. An elderly woman sat beside me on my left, and then a Hispanic man around my age sat on the corner to her left. The services began, and I felt the Holy Spirit tugging at my heart.

When the pastor began his sermon, every word out of his mouth sounded as if he was electronically attached to my brain. I began to weep. The more he preached, the more he touched on subjects heavy on my heart, and the weeping intensified. I felt like I had a direct line to God. The pastor finished his sermon, he then blessed and released us. I waited for the elderly woman to exit and then I noticed the Hispanic man waiting at the pew's end. I approached him.

He offered his hand, introduced himself, and asked me how I was doing.

I told him, "You would not believe what I have been through and am going through now!"

His response was: "Everything's going to be all right. The Holy Spirit told me to tell you, 'EVERYTHING YOU'RE PRAYING FOR WILL COME TO PASS.'"

I immediately felt the joy and love of the Lord. I thanked the man repeatedly and went on my way. While on my way home, I decided to call my mother and tell her about my experience. During my conversation I began to weep profusely, just as I am doing right now while writing this chapter. That night, I called my brother and Jessica to tell them what happened. Both were overjoyed.

Another milestone in my spiritual awakening was a sermon regarding tithing and wave-offerings. The pastor had two bundles of what appeared to be wheat grass—one was thick green and beautifully bundled, and the other was, bundled carelessly, and was gangly and somewhat dried-out. His question to us was: "Which would you rather present to our Lord?"

This struck home with me, and it made me rethink my tithing practices. I began to examine how I could afford to give more to the Lord. This sounds totally ridiculous to me now, because my thought process now is: "How will I survive without my tithe and offering?" Shortly after that sermon, I had a dream. When I woke up, I could not remember the dream, but I remembered a bible verse from the dream. I'm embarrassed to tell you this now, but I had to search for my bible in order to look up that verse. Once I found it, I hurriedly looked up the scripture. I don't remember the exact chapter and verse, but I believe it was in the book of Deuteronomy, and the verse basically said this: "Do not come into the house of the Lord empty-handed." The Lord was telling me he wanted to bless me, but I wasn't following the rules in the right manner. After this, I made sure I never went to church without an offering. Whatever was leftover was what I brought.

Now a person mature in the spirit would read that last sentence and say, "Wrong, wrong, wrong!" I am still maturing in the spirit, and I now practice *First Fruits*. I was doing the right thing by tithing;

but I was just doing it in the wrong order. Let me elaborate as well as I can on the subject of First Fruits. This means putting God first—in your life, in your finances, and in all aspects of your life. The first check I write after a deposit is to my church, and then I begin my bill-paying process. Even when the enemy is telling me, "You don't have enough money to write that check; you should apply those funds to another bill you have," I simply shout, "The devil is a liar! My God provides and sustains me, for he is the Almighty. No one is greater than he who lives within me!"

Putting God first by sowing that seed into the rich ground of heaven puts you into a position of favor with the Lord. Isn't that what all Christians are looking for? I'm telling you, it's working for me, but I do not look for instant gratification. God constantly tests our faith, but remember God is always faithful. He has removed me from some tough experiences in life; some examples of which are noted in earlier chapters. I cannot impress upon you the importance of First Fruits Tithes, and offerings. For example, I had two years of slow to nonexistent business. This was during my wrong-tithing times, and this put me in debt to the tune of thirty thousand dollars, not including house and car. When I started practicing the principals of First Fruits, it took ten months to reap a harvest, but when I did, was it ever a blessing! I was about three months behind on bills! Had this enormous debt staring me in the face, and I owed around six thousand in back taxes. A lot of people would have considered personal bankruptcy, but not me. I held onto my faith. Within a year and a half, I reduced my debt to eleven thousand, and my taxes and bills were current. If that wasn't divine intervention, then I do not know what is.

# (7) RESULTS

Through all of the aforementioned trials and tribulations, I have watched myself mature spiritually, and I have witnessed the need for God in my life growing by leaps and bounds. I'm not quite where he wants me positioned yet, but I plan on getting there as quickly as I can. The first thing I must do is shed this worldly skin and replace it with one that is heaven-sent, which requires removing myself from positions of temptation. I have found that temptation is rarely manifested when avoidance is implemented!

Prior to attending Cornerstone, my prayer life was little to nonexistent. I was what my pastor calls a "crisis Christian." I only prayed after I had exhausted all my efforts for resolving the issue or problem. After reading previous chapters, a lot of you readers are probably thinking, "As much as this guy has been through, he must have been praying constantly." Then there are those of you who have read between the lines and realize how stubborn I can be and understand how I tried to fix the problems myself, with little result. I am better-educated in the spirit now, and I know which direction to turn for guidance and help.

I spoke in earlier chapters about some of the blessings I have received. I would like to elaborate on those somewhat now. Around five years ago, I received my final settlement from my ex-wife, and for a man who has lived most of his life in the lower-middle-class section, this was a pretty good chunk of change. My first thought was to give my church ten percent, and I did. The blessings I received that year were ten-fold. For example, the average size of jobs I had been obtaining was between three and five thousand dollars. This was the year I landed the patio enclosure in early spring, then the whole house-remodel in late fall. Each of these jobs were in the fifteen-thousand-dollar range. See how the Lord strategically spread them out to sustain me? Glory to his name! The New Year of 2005 was looking pretty bleak, due to the latter half of 2004 being pretty slow, but I kept seeing hope in this New Year, and I promised God that, no matter what, I would tithe regularly. As I mentioned earlier, the blessings were phenomenal. They took ten months to arrive, but they were welcomed with opened arms. God puts us in these situations to allow us to draw closer to him. I thank him daily for these hardships.

Around the middle of year 2005, when business was pretty dreary, I began to ponder what I was still doing wrong. It became apparent that my prayer life was still lacking, even though I prayed on a much more regular basis now. I began to reposition myself by devoting a certain amount of time each morning, before I start my day, to praise and worship. There were also a few silent moments during the day. During the evening, I began to immerse myself in the Word. All of this brought joy and peace to my tumultuous life.

That same year took me out of town for work. I knew this job would take several weeks, and late in the week, I started to become frantic. How was I going to worship on Sunday? It was too far to drive back and forth, or at least I thought so. I began to pray about this issue on Saturday night, asking God's forgiveness for my delinquency. I promised I would spend at least an hour in prayer and worship. I woke up the next morning, turned on the television, then jumped into the shower. As I was making my way out of the shower, I heard my pastor's booming voice coming from the television. I jumped with joy. It was almost as good as being there! I quickly dressed while my eyes were glued to the screen. My eyes began to well up with joy, for the Lord knew I needed a little piece of home, and he sustained me again. I noted the time and channel for next week.

Don't you find it amazing how little things like that always seem to happen to those who maintain their faith? I think back on times that seemed somewhat coincidental, and I realize how much divine intervention has been performed throughout my life. For instance, my dream with the scripture which pertained to tithing, noted in a previous chapter. No one can attribute that to anything other than divine intervention. My stroke-recovery was nothing short of a miracle! Earlier in my childhood, I survived a horrendous car accident at the ripe old age of ten. My injuries include a fractured skull in two places and a concussion. My upper lip was almost cut off; it was hanging by a piece of skin about a quarter-inch long. My head was swollen to the size of a bowling ball. This accident also happened in October, so I guess you can say I'm not terribly fond of the month of October. After an extensive stay in a local hospital, I returned to normal activities such as school and church. When our pastor's wife saw me at church my first time since the accident, she told my mother, "God has something planned for that little boy!" That has stuck in my head since 1969.

Another incident involving a vehicle was during my teenage years. While driving home from work late one evening during a very heavy rain, I became a little disoriented, made a wrong turn, and ended up sideways in a ditch that was flowing with rain water. Water began to fill my car. I quickly scrambled out the passenger door, which was no easy task, since the car was at about a forty-five-degree angle. The full weight of the door had to be pushed straight up and held in place while I got out. Then I walked about three miles home in the pouring rain, but God sustained me.

One other time, while tubing the Guadalupe with my wife and other friends, I failed to veer left and get out and walk around the bridge at Gruene. Water was right at the bottom of the bridge. The current slammed me into the bridge. I tried to climb up onto the bridge, but I lost my grip and was swept under. Then my legs became tangled in some brush or tree limbs. I struggled and fought until I freed myself, then floated out into calmer waters. Would you call this coincidence or divine intervention? I believe the latter of the two, and hope you do, also.

There have been too many instances in my life and way too many close calls, not to attribute it to the work of the Lord. If you are a non-believer or just have drifted away from the Lord, just ask his forgiveness for your sins. Repent, and ask him to come into your life. He's calling your name right now;

He misses you and wants you back in his protected flock. Can you hear his loving call? Try listening with your heart, then reach out to him. He is waiting with open arms. Can you hear your name? He is calling. Please don't turn a deaf ear to our savior. He loves you and has many great things in store for you. Now let's try it again: open your heart, and I'm sure you can hear His plea

If you are truly committed to radical change in your life, after you allow him into your heart, you will begin to hunger and thirst for righteousness with a passion. I find myself praying five or six times a day, and on difficult days, much more than that. I also watch television evangelists on a regular basis now. The funny thing about that is, I always receive a message that, whether direct or implied, impacts my situation in some way, shape, or form. Most of the time, it seems as if that person is speaking directly to me about my issues and problems, which makes me feel like God is telling me, "I know what you're going through. Just persevere, and everything will be all right." This brings peace and comfort to me.

# (8) REVELATION

Just to give you a little insight on my personality, I have a daily quota of making five people smile or laugh. I've been doing this for six years now, and have never missed a smile or laugh quota. I believe laughter is a healthy benefit in our Christian lives. I try to laugh as often as I can. I receive a genuine thrill when I can brighten up someone's day—actually, I feel blessed. It is amazing how well people respond when you show small acts of kindness. Try it, and you will be surprised. They will open up to you, and who knows? They might even attempt the process on the next person they meet. Can you imagine a world where everyone attempts to make each person they meet smile or laugh? It sounds kind of like Heaven on Earth to me. Jesus did not willingly shed his blood on the cross so that the majority of us can be irate and short-tempered. Jesus willingly gave the ultimate sacrifice of death on the cross so we can enjoy eternal life. Should we repay him with hate and discontent? I believe small acts of kindness are a necessary component for maturing spiritually. Don't get me wrong: I'm not saying random acts of kindness will get you into Heaven. All I'm saying is that I would find it extremely difficult as a practicing Christian not to display these acts on a daily basis.

I have often sat and dreamed about this woman the Lord has promised me; all right I have fantasized about her. What color is her hair? How tall is she? Does she have children? Is her faith so much greater that mine is challenged daily, possibly hourly? I would readily greet a challenge of this sort. I can't wait until we can rise together early one frosty, winter morning, grab a huge blanket, and snuggle together on a patio bench, engaged in stimulating conversation and anxiously awaiting sunrise—or just relax on a beach or at the lake, watching the sun go down, while reflecting on our surroundings and verbally washing each other with compliments and praise. Common, everyday occurrences such as conversing with your spouse about your day is an event most people take for granted. Most of you do not realize how difficult it is to come home to an empty house every day, prepare your dinner sit-down, and eat alone. That is when the feeling of loneliness is so overwhelming and unbearable at times, I am literally dying inside for my phone to ring and bring a small amount of comfort to my otherwise tumultuous and lonely life. Anticipation of returning home daily and finding someone I care about and who also cares about me is all I live and breathe for!

Simple activities, such as the aforementioned sunrise-sunset, are of utmost importance to me and things I yearn for daily. I'm sure the companionship that this woman will bring into my life will make the last ten years fade, just as the sunset fades.

I have even thought how, after a year or so, or ten or more years of marriage, we would be relaxing one evening while watching television, and my attention would turn to just gazing upon her. After an extended amount of time, she would notice me looking at her and ask, "What are you doing?"

I would reply, "Just trying to forget what life was like without you, and I am just in awe of your grace, charm, and beauty!"

She responds, "You're so sweet." Then she casually approaches and embraces me with the strength of an N.F.L linebacker, which of course, is followed by a soft kiss, loving conversation, and adoration. I can't wait until I find this woman the lord has promised. Who knows? Maybe she will buy this book and start searching for me! Maybe that's what the Lord had planned all along.

Nevertheless, I still wait in anticipation of finally meeting this divine example of a woman. Until the Lord reveals her to me, I must remain content with dreaming about her and our Garden of Eden.

I hope you have enjoyed my story, it was extremely difficult at times stirring that pot again, but if anyone can benefit from this, it was well worth the trouble. My thanks, and God's blessings to all of you.